Forever Amen

Forever. Amen
Copyright © 2021 Nathan Lyle Cunningham. All rights reserved.

All rights reserved. No part of this publication may be reproduced, stored in a retrieval system, or transmitted in any way by any means – electronic, mechanical, photocopy, recording, or otherwise – without the prior permissions of the copyright holder, except by reviewer who may quote brief passages in a review to be printed in magazine newspaper or by radio / TV announcement, as provided by USA copyright law. The author and the publisher will not be held responsible for any errors within the manuscript. All characters appearing in this work are fictitious. Any resemblance to real persons, living or dead, is purely coincidental. Unless otherwise indicated, all scripture quotations are taken from the King James Version of the Bible.

F I R S T   E D I T I O N
Published in 2021

Author: Nathan Lyle Cunningham
www.YouTube.com/NathanLyleOfficial
www.Twitter.com/NathanLyle

ISBN: 978-1-7343061-2-5

Library of Congress in Publication Data

Category: Family, Relationships, Social

Library of Congress Cataloging-in-Publication Data

Publishing Consultant & Designer: Eli Blyden | EliTheBookGuy.com

Printed & Published in the United States of America

* * *

Dying is the easy part.
It's the people left behind that really suffer.

* * *

Forever. Amen

Table of Contents

CHAPTER 1
Trevor 1

CHAPTER 2
Amanda 11

CHAPTER 3
Melanie 19

CHAPTER 4
Traci 27

CHAPTER 5
Amanda 33

CHAPTER 6
Melanie 37

CHAPTER 7
Cynthia 41

CHAPTER 8
Amanda 49

CHAPTER 9
Trevor 55

CHAPTER 10
Melanie 61

CHAPTER 11
Amanda 67

Other Books by Nathan Lyle Cunningham 71

Forever. Amen

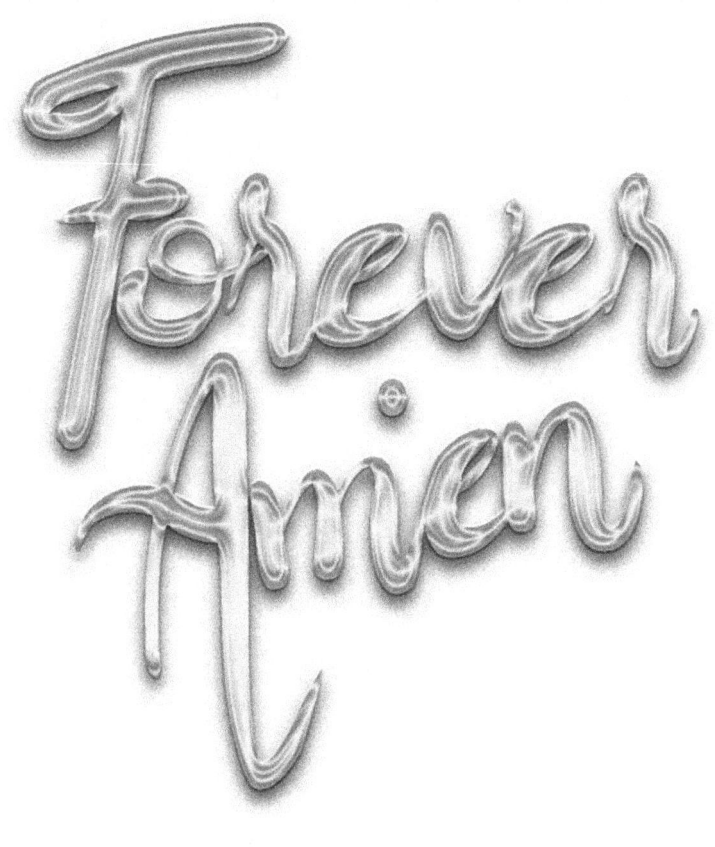

BY NATHAN LYLE CUNNINGHAM

Forever. Amen

CHAPTER 1

Trevor

Fall has always been my favorite time of year. The days were warm but only mildly. No one actually broke a sweat. As the sun set a cool breeze swept through the city bringing a feeling of freshness to the air.

On a Sunday night in the middle of September the six of us gathered at the restaurant Aurora. We liked to call it the snow globe. It was a circular building. The walls were panels of glass stood side by side and stacked on top of each other. We loved going there at night so we could see the moon through the ceiling.

The only section of the restaurant that wasn't transparent was the bar. A wooden wall that took up maybe a fifth of the building. Shelves stacked about eight feet high, loaded with wine, beer and liquor. In front of that wall was an L-shaped counter. On a busy night you could see as many as five bartenders frantically trying to keep up with the orders. That night, with a half empty dining room, there were only two of them back there leisurely mixing drinks.

Off to the side was a rectangular opening covered by two thin black curtains that stopped inches above the ground.

From time to time the curtains parted as bodies passed through. A server carried out plates of food. A busser carried dirty dishes back into the room. A cook walked out to greet a table.

The six of us were at a circular table furthest from that curtain. I sat with my back to the room. The cityscape at night was a far more enjoyable sight than strangers stuffing their faces. Not that I'm much to look at either.

Just under six feet tall with mahogany skin that matched the floorboards beneath our feet. Just enough curly black hair to cover the top of my head. I never paid much attention to fashion. My clothes were always oversized to hide the protruding belly and underarm flab.

I never let my nails grow too long. I constantly bit them. I know it's not healthy but I couldn't stop myself if I tried. The moment I notice my nails have grown past the tips of my fingers my teeth promptly clamp down on them.

Our table was the loudest in the restaurant. I did my best to minimize the noise pollution by sparsely participating in the conversation. I slightly raised the corners of my mouth in an effort to convince them that I actually wanted to be there when really I'd rather be back home, sitting on my couch watching the game.

There was one reason why I stayed amidst the gaggle. One reason why, from time to time, the forced smile on my face was replaced by a real one. That reason's name was Melanie Rios. A few inches above five feet. Round brown eyes that always twinkled. Wavy chestnut hair that fell down her lightly bronzed shoulders. Round lips coated by a layer of gloss.

She always took care of her body. Ate her vegetables; exercised daily. She was never the type to have pounds of makeup caked on her face but that day there was more color than usual. I don't think I ever saw her in a dress. Not that I mind. She looked amazing in jeans. That thin blue blouse didn't hurt either.

For most of the night her head was on a swivel, careful to give each person attention. Occasionally, she would look my way. Just long enough to make sure I was still there. Every time her head turned my way my smile widened.

Sitting on Melanie's right was her cousin Amanda. She's relatively tall, only a couple of inches shorter than me, wearing a short black skirt and a matching jacket over a red tank top. A large hoop dangled from each earlobe. She ran her long, thin fingers through her long, thin black hair. Everything about her is long and thin. Her arms, legs and neck. Her nose, eyes and lips. Long and thin with caramel skin.

She always has a magisterial air about her. Many people, myself included, have trouble getting along with her. She doesn't go out of her way to insult you. She just doesn't dance around the truth to protect your feelings. Getting used to her can be a struggle but the frankness soon becomes her most endearing quality.

To Melanie's left sat her younger sister Traci. They're similar enough that many strangers mistake them for twins. The most obvious differences are that Traci is a little taller with lighter skin, darker hair and rounder features. Would it be mean to say that she's like an overinflated Melanie balloon?

I counted twenty piercings on her ears. The lack of symmetry bothered me. There were thirteen on her right ear and seven on her left. Every outfit she's ever worn included a low cut top and a pair of combat boots. There's very little wear and tear. It's safe to assume that they're nothing more than a fashion statement and not meant for real world application.

Sitting between Traci and I was Amanda's older sister Cynthia. Funny enough, Traci's hair looked more like Amanda's while Cynthia's hair looked more like Melanie's. Her hair and skin had the lightest tones of anyone at this table. I don't want to say she was overdressed but her navy blue dress and matching heels definitely stood out compared to the overall casual feel of the table.

I had very few personal interactions with Cynthia. She appeared every now and then to offer a clever quip intermingled with some words of wisdom. She always maintained a certain level of emotional detachment.

Sitting between Amanda and I was Amanda's boyfriend Zack. He'd only been a part of the group for a few months. I know I shouldn't compare myself to others but it's impossible to look at a man like him and not feel inferior. You look up chiseled in the dictionary and you'll see a picture of his body. Even I have to admit that he's unbelievably cute.

I never asked him what he did for a living. I assumed he was a marine. When I think of the marines, people like him are what come to mind. I never saw him in anything other than cargo pants and a t-shirt. Even all his shorts were cargo. Half the time his shirts were so tight you could see every single muscle on his abdomen. He definitely did that on purpose.

If it was my choice I never would've said a single word to him. Unfortunately, since I was the only other guy in our group he actively sought out my company. Too bad our similar physiology is the only commonality we shared. If we were coworkers this is the kind of guy I would smile and make small talk with but always turn down every time he invited me out for a drink after work.

We ate a full course meal, complete with wine and cocktails, conversing for hours before the group began to disperse. Amanda and Zack left first, walking out the door hand in hand as the remaining members speculated about how the two of them would spend their last waking hours of the night.

"I guarantee you Mandy is always on top. She's too much of a control freak to just lie there doing nothing the entire time."

"You're totally wrong. Mandy definitely likes it doggy. That way she can read while she waits for him to finish."

Since my experience in that area is limited the only insight I could offer was a cleverly thought out rebuttal that canceled out all their theories. Devil's advocate seemed to be my primary function in most conversations.

"You're all operating under the assumption that they actually have sex. For all we know he could be a eunuch. Have any of you ever seen his penis?"

"Yes."

We all whipped our heads to stare at Melanie. Traci seemed shocked. Cynthia seemed curious. Me...I felt my heart sinking and stomach churning. My entire body was filled with immense dread. I tried my best not to let it show.

"What," Melanie chuckled, "He sent Mandy a picture and she showed me."

I sighed in relief and slumped back down in my chair.

"How was it?"

"Not that big. But at least he keeps it shaved."

I pulled out my phone to look at the time.

"It's getting late. I'm gonna head home."

I slid my phone back into my pocket as I rose from my chair. When Melanie saw me standing she hurried to her feet.

"I'll give you a ride home."

She always jumped at the chance to drive me somewhere. Partly because I used not having a car as an excuse not to go out much. If she didn't offer to pick me up we'd spend half as much time together.

I don't mind a pedestrian lifestyle. Number one rule of finding a place to live: location, location, location. My job is only a half hour walk from my apartment. There are multiple stores and fast food places within that thirty minute radius. Plus, traveling on physical power is the only reason I stay under three hundred pounds. I'll never be skinny but at least I avoid obesity.

All that said, I cherished every moment spent in Melanie's passenger seat. The window down; a breeze in my face.

Neither of us said a word. I didn't mind. I was happy just being near her.

She was always smiling. I never saw anything close to a frown on her face. Some days I wished I could see her cry just to make sure she was a normal human. Being around someone who's always cheerful is too intimidating.

She glanced my way every time we stopped at a light. Even when her head wasn't pointed directly at me I could tell that she was looking at me out of the corner of her eye.

I wanted to say something. Anything. Something to make her laugh. Something to make her cry. Something to make her ponder the mysteries of the universe. My mouth just wouldn't move. We stopped at another red light and she turned her head to me.

"Your apartment's a one bedroom right?"

"Yeah."

"Any chance you'd let me stay the night?"

My heart was beating like a jackhammer. I could barely breathe.

"Why would you want to?"

"Save's time. And gas money."

"My bed's not big enough for two."

"Not even if I sleep on top of you?"

My heart skipped a beat. My head filled with images of her and I laying in each other's arms under the covers. I took a deep breath, trying to calm myself down as I wiggled around in my seat turning my knees towards the door.

"I have a couch."

"You can't make a girl sleep on the couch."

"You can't kick me out of my own bed."

"I said we can share."

I hoped she was teasing me. There's no man on this planet with the restraint to share a bed with any female, even one he isn't interested in, without making a move. If she was being serious that meant she didn't see me as a man. I was another one of her girlfriends.

We rolled to a stop in front of my apartment complex and I rushed to unbuckle my seatbelt. As my hand moved to unlock the door I felt her hand on my shoulder.

"I'm sorry. I wasn't trying to upset you."

I turned my head back to her. No one could doubt her sincerity when looking into those eyes.

"It's ok. I'm good."

That same familiar smile spread across her face as she reached down to unbuckle her seatbelt. She leaned forward with her arms outstretched. I leaned towards her and wrapped my arms around her torso while she wrapped her arms around my neck.

Her body was so slender I could feel every single one of her ribs. A few strands of her hair fell in front of my face. I inhaled deeply. As her scent filled my nose a warm sensation flowed through my body. I pulled her closer. She giggled and tightened her grip. We stayed like that for a few seconds before pulling away.

We sat there a few more seconds staring at each other with smiles on our faces. For a moment, just a brief moment,

I wondered what would happen if I leaned in for a kiss. Would my attempt be met with joy and excitement? No. More than likely the feeling of my lips against hers would cause dismay and disdain.

"Goodnight."

"Goodnight."

I swung the door open and jumped out. As I slammed the door shut she gave me one last wave goodbye. I waved back. She buckled her seat belt and drove off. I took a deep breath, held it for a couple of seconds, then exhaled. I walked towards the front door knowing I would need a long, cold shower before I went to bed.

Forever. Amen

CHAPTER 2

Amanda

The two of us sat in the doctor's office. It was a small room, maybe eighty or ninety square feet. Melanie and I sat in the middle of the room on two wooden chairs with cushioned seats. The door was behind us. On the wall in front of us was a small window. The blinds were down but through the tilted slats I could see the leaves on the branch of a nearby tree.

There were two bookcases, one on each side wall. Both of them overstuffed with what I can only assume are textbooks and medical journals. There were three degrees on his wall. No wonder doctors cost so much. They're trying to pay back those college loans.

There was a wooden desk in front of us with a few things scattered on top. A closed laptop, a notepad and a couple of pens. A half empty cup of coffee. My eyes were drawn to the picture of three children standing next to each other. A girl on the right and the other two both boys.

The boy in the middle was the tallest. Couldn't have been more than ten years old. I wondered what his name might be.

Looked like a Kevin. Maybe a Joseph. If I had a son what would I name him? I've always liked Emanuel.

I turned my head to look at Melanie. I'll never understand morning people. How is it possible for anyone to wake up in the morning and spend two hours on hair and makeup? When I go out at night I'll try my best but for early mornings I'll do the bare minimum I need to make myself not ugly.

Melanie's mouth would not stop moving. Sometimes she amazed me. If I asked Melanie a question about herself she'd respond with one word answers. Yet any time Trevor was mentioned she'd drone on for hours.

"Are you fucking serious?"

I hate that habit of mine. The words fly out of my mouth immediately after the thought enters my head. It makes it hard to keep people in my life. Then again, it's really easy to chase away people I can't stand.

"How long have you two been together now? Two years? Just fuck already."

"We're not dating. We're just…really good friends."

"He goes grocery shopping with you. If you asked him to marry you he'd definitely say yes. Hell, that guy would carry your babies."

"You mean he'd ask me to carry his babies?"

"I said what I meant."

Melanie looked at me with a face that very few on this planet have ever seen. A face that combines anger and sadness into a look of disappointment that seems almost exclusively reserved for me and Traci.

"What do you like about that guy anyways?"

"He's one of the sweetest, most caring people I've ever met."

"If you love him so much why not ask him out?"

"I won't push him into anything that he's not ready for."

"What if he never ask you out? He's such a pussy."

"He actually stops to think about other people's feelings. Unlike some cousins I have."

"At this rate you're both gonna die alone."

"At least we'll die alone together."

I turned around in my chair when I heard the door swing open. Dr. Lewis walked in the room and pulled the door closed behind him. He was a tall, middle-aged man who always had bags under his eyes. Short black hair with gray strands scattered around. As he walked past my chair I noticed a folder in his hands.

He walked around to the other side of the desk and sat in the swiveling black chair. He cleared his throat, dropped the file on his desk and opened it. After staring down at it silently for a few seconds he took a deep breath and looked up at Melanie. That look made my heart race. It made my stomach churn. It's a look I've seen on far too many faces.

The first time I saw that look I was eight years old. Dr. Maylock told my parents that Melanie's father was working at a construction site when a steel beam fell on him. He bled to death before the ambulance arrived. Two years later my parents had that look on their faces when they sat Cynthia and I down to tell us that Melanie's mom was dying of cancer.

It's the same look I saw on Dr. Jeremiah's face when I was twenty. She told me my parents were in a car crash. My father died immediately on impact. They tried to save my mom but she had too many internal injuries. Five years later Doctor Sowell had the same look on her face when she told us my sister was HIV positive.

When I saw Dr. Lewis staring at Melanie with that same look on his face I tilted my head up to the ceiling, searching the clouds for any sign of omniscience. Feeling relieved when I found none.

I can accept that this might be some random roll of the dice and my life just happened to come up snake eyes. If you try to tell me this is part of some convoluted plan I might punch you in the face. What kind of inane plan would require me to endure so much pain?

"Thank you for coming so early. I'm sorry we kept you waiting."

"No problem."

"What's this all about? Is something wrong with Melanie?"

Melanie placed a hand on my shoulder. Her way of telling me, "down girl. Don't bite the nice doctor." When I leaned back in my chair she pulled her hand away. Dr. Lewis sighed and ran his fingers through his hair.

"If it's ok with you, I want to ask you some questions about your medical history. Double check some things."

"That's fine."

"So, you only visit the doctor once a year to get your annual physical? No major injuries or illnesses that required extended hospital stays?"

"I've stayed in a few hospitals, just not as a patient. The worst I've ever gotten was a cold that kept me in bed for two days."

"During your exam you mentioned breathing problems. When did you first notice that?"

"Um, A few months I think. But it's not too bad. It only hurts when I'm exercising."

"Have you noticed anything else? Fatigue? Loss of appetite?"

"Yeah, but...I figured all of that was cause I stopped working out."

The doctor lowered his head, taking slow, deep breaths before looking back at Melanie with somber eyes.

"How much do you know about your mother's death?"

I looked at Melanie. Her eyes were wide, as if staring through the darkness, searching for some ray of hope. I knew she was waiting for me to say something kind and encouraging but I couldn't find the words.

I knew that if I started freaking out she would as well. I tried my best to keep my breathing steady. My heart was trying to break through my chest but I couldn't let her see that. I grabbed my knee and squeezed it while grinding my teeth.

"My mom died from cancer."

"Do you remember the specific type?"

"I, um...n-n-no, I, I, I..."

"Small cell carcinoma."

Melanie and Dr. Lewis both turned their heads to me.

"I never understood what the words meant. I know it has something to do with her lungs."

The doctor nodded twice before turning back to Melanie.

"Since it's in your medical records it's something we've always kept a look out for. Unfortunately, it seems we've found it."

Melanie extended her arm and I grabbed her trembling hand. It was like grabbing a skeleton. Were her fingers always so skinny? Oh my god…is this my fault? Should I have seen the signs?

"I'm afraid the news doesn't stop there. Your carcinoma has reached extensive stage."

"What does that mean?"

"In simplest terms, it's moved beyond the lungs."

Melanie tightened her grip. It hurt a bit. I stroked her fingers with my thumb.

"What can we do?"

"Platinum based combination chemotherapy is the standard of care. However, I do need to inform you that even in cases where a patient is declared cancer free, a relapse can occur. With extensive-stage, the long-term survival rate is incredibly low. That being said, if you do nothing at all the chance of survival is virtually zero. I recommend we begin treatment as soon as humanly possible."

I knew that I needed to keep my composure. I had to stay strong for Melanie's sake. I had to show her that she could lean on me. I failed. The moment I saw tears rolling down her cheeks I felt them falling out of my eyes as well.

Forever. Amen

CHAPTER 3

Melanie

I lived in a quaint little house with my sister and cousins. A one floor building with a kitchen, living room, bathroom and 3 bedrooms. Technically there's only one bedroom but when we bought the place Amanda said, "You can turn any room into bedroom. Just throw a mattress in there."

The two smaller rooms were barely big enough to squeeze a twin bed into. Barely any leg room. Even less breathing room. The sole benefit of those rooms is the ability to completely isolate yourself. Once the door was closed everyone left you alone.

The master bedroom was the worst place to be if you wanted to sleep late. It's the most comfortable bed but it's also the biggest so you'll usually end up sharing it with at least one other person. Not to mention that room had the only closet in the house. We also shoved the dresser in there.

Nearly every piece of clothing that existed in the house resided in that room. Most days people would at least try to be quiet and tiptoe around but there have been some incredibly turbulent exceptions.

I spent the afternoon on the big bed, laying on top of the comforter with my phone resting on the pillow in front of me. Since we got back from the hospital I spent the day scrolling through pictures on my phone; digging through every single social media platform, looking at every photo I could find of my friends and family.

Time is an amazing thing. I spent most of my life wondering why the clock was so slow. Spent every day wondering how much longer it would be. How much longer before this day ends and I get to go home? How many more years of torture before I'm finally done with school for good?

Then one day I thought about my teen years and six years of puberty all blended together. Did I get my septum pierced at fifteen or sixteen? No, I was 17 and it was my belly button. I didn't pierce my nose till I was nineteen. Then I took it out a week later. It got on my nerves.

A lifetime of memories, some of which I hadn't thought about since they happened, were all popping into my head. It was bittersweet. My short life could be coming to an abrupt end. I wouldn't be able to make any more memories.

I heard the *clunk clunk* of Amanda's boots stomping towards me. I never understood how someone so skinny could have such heavy footsteps. She stepped in the door so fast I could almost feel a breeze. She leaned against the door frame and crossed her arms.

"Everyone's here."

I pushed the power button on my phone and slid it into my pocket.

"I don't wanna tell the family."

"Isn't that the whole reason we told them to come here?"

"Not them. I mean all of our aunts, uncles and cousins. I don't want any of them to know."

"You want me to kick Traci and Cynthia out?"

I rolled my eyes.

"There's a difference. We see them every day. Even if we say nothing they'll still realize something is wrong."

I swung my legs around and slid down to the edge of the bed.

"I know every single relative I have would put their entire life on hold to be there for me if I asked them to. But that would only make me feel guilty."

Amanda dropped down to her knees directly in front of me.

"It's important to have family by your side when you're going through troubled times."

"What can they do? Pray for me?"

"What's gotten into you?"

"I don't want them to know. Why is that wrong?"

"What if you don't make it? Don't they deserve the chance to say goodbye?"

"Well maybe that's why I don't want them here. Maybe seeing the despair on their faces will make it harder to keep my hopes up. Maybe I'm not ready to accept my death yet."

I was trying to hold them back but I could feel the teardrops falling. I lifted my arms to wipe my eyes but before I could Amanda grabbed my hands.

"And maybe being surrounded by people you love makes it easier to fight."

I adjusted the position of my hands so I could give hers a good squeeze.

"I already have plenty to fight for."

She closed her eyes and lowered her head. I kissed the top of her head. Most people believe that Amanda has no filter. They'd be shocked if they found out how much she actually held back. At that moment she probably wanted to ignore everything I said and tell the family everything.

"Well...you are the one with cancer. It's your choice whether or not you tell people."

I placed a hand on her cheek.

"Thank you."

Amanda took a deep breath and let out a huge sigh. She jumped to her feet and left the room. A few seconds later she walked back in with a wad of toilet paper.

"We've really gotta start keeping tissues in this house."

Amanda wiped my face dry then held the wad under my nose.

"Blow."

She wiped my nose and threw the dirty wad in the waste basket. Then she stood in front of me and held out her hand.

"Come on. Everyone's waiting."

I dropped my hands in hers and gripped them firmly. With one yank she pulled me to my feet and led me out the door. I don't know if it's her long stride or my anxieties but being pulled along behind her almost felt like someone tied me to the back of a car and drove away at two hundred miles an hour. Hell, that might've be slightly less painful than making the announcement.

No one who saw our house could possibly mistake us for interior decorators. The living room had just enough furniture to suit our needs. A grey two-seat sofa pressed against one wall. On the opposite wall, a foot from the front door, a twenty inch smart TV rested on a small table with a wood top and metal frame.

There was a coffee table in front of the sofa. Not big enough for a thanksgiving feast but we could comfortably fit four plates on there. On both sides of the sofa were cheap plastics chairs that we threw comforters over and tossed some pillows onto.

Near the wall furthest from the door was the captain's chair. That's the name we gave to a blue recliner that, for tiny bodies like ours, could double as a bed. It had the worst view of the TV but it was the most comfortable place to sit in the entire building. You could always tell who showed up first just by looking at that chair.

Cynthia was in the captain's chair, fully reclined with her eyes glued to her phone. Traci was sprawled out across the sofa, her feet dangling off the end, holding her phone above her face. Trevor and Zack were sitting in the chairs. Zack was staring at the ceiling while Trevor sullenly stared at the floor. When we walked in the room Amanda cleared her throat and everyone raised their heads.

"I'm sure you're all wondering why I called you here."

"You're pregnant! Congrats!"

Traci playfully patted Zack's knee. Amanda rolled her eyes.

"Can you ever take anything seriously?"

"I promise to take your pregnancy very seriously."

"I seriously wish I wasn't related to you."

"Same."

While Amanda and Traci had their pissing contest I crossed my arms and leaned back against the wall. Trevor's refused to take his eyes off me. The look on his face suggested that he could tell something was wrong. He rose to his feet and took steps towards me.

As he approached I felt my heartbeat quickening. The fear of having to say the words out loud had me on the edge of hyperventilation. He stopped a few inches in front of me. He stood there staring, his brown eyes piercing deep into my soul. I couldn't stop the tears. Cynthia and Traci both sat upright.

"Melanie has been diagnosed with Cancer."

Shock, dismay, concern and overwhelming sadness. That's what I read on each of their faces. Traci's mouth was on the floor. Cynthia slumped back in the chair. She looked like she was trying to decide whether to cry or punch something.

Zack had the same sympathetic look on his face that most people would give to a four year old lost in the mall crying for her mommy. Trevor went out of his way to keep a stone face but I could see the tears welling up in his eyes.

"What kind of cancer?"

"Extensive-stage small cell carcinoma."

Cynthia clutched her chest. A feeling of despair swept over the room. Traci raised her head to look at me.

"What does that mean?"

She reminded me of a child, looking at me with those round eyes like she didn't understand why her fish is swimming upside down.

"It means she's going to die."

When Cynthia said those words it felt like a sword made of ice was shoved into my heart.

"We don't know that for sure."

"It's the exact same thing that killed her mom."

"That doesn't guarantee Melanie won't make it."

"Both of you shut up."

That surprised me. I've never heard Trevor yell. His voice was so booming it left an echo. I straightened up and swallow a lump in my throat.

"I have cancer."

Wow. I actually said it. The words sounded so normal but felt so heavy.

"What's the survival rate?"

"Incredibly low."

"But it's more than zero?"

I nodded. He leaned forward and whispered, "Then there's hope." It was amazing. As much as Trevor and Amanda hated each other they had one important thing in common. They always seemed to know exactly how to calm me down. I wrapped my arms around his stomach and rested my head on his chest. The rhythm of his heart soothed me. He wrapped one arm around my shoulders and rested his other hand on my head.

CHAPTER 4

Traci

Most days I preferred driving with the windows down so I could feel the breeze. As the temperature dropped the cold wind started feeling like little knives jabbing my face. Once winter began the windows were always up and the heater was always on.

Melanie was asleep in the passenger seat. It was the first time we'd ever been in a car together without her yelling at me. She and Amanda look for any excuse to remind me of all the bad decisions I've made in my life.

Pulling up to the house felt different. A week after we moved in I was already tired of that place. I would gladly jump at any excuse to not be there. After Melanie was diagnosed with cancer I spent every possible second there.

"Hey. Wake- up."

I nudged her gently as I whispered to her. She groaned and wriggled in her seat. I nudged her again. She waved me away and mumbled something.

"Wake! Up!"

Melanie reluctantly opened her eyes and stretched out her arms and legs.

"Are we in the car?"
"Yup."
"I fell asleep again?"
"Yeah."
"I'm sorry."
"It's fine. I drive better when you're not yelling at me."

We got out of the car and went inside. The moment I swung the door open the smell of cheeseburgers wafted towards me. I tilted my head to peek in the kitchen and saw Trevor. I've never been a huge fan of the guy but I'm willing to accept him as a member of the family if it means I get to eat his cooking once in a while.

Amanda and Zack were sitting on the sofa with their fingers interlocked. When we walked in the room Amanda tapped Zack's knee and he stood up and moved to the chair. When Melanie sat in the vacated spot Amanda threw an arm around Melanie's shoulder and kissed her forehead.

"You feeling ok?"
"Yeah. I'm fine."

Trevor walked in the room holding two small bowls filled with vegetables and put them on the table in front of Melanie and Amanda.

"What is this?"

As he walked out of the room Trevor yells, "It's a Spinach and broccoli salad with roasted almonds and grilled chicken."

"But why though?"
"Amanda told me to."

Melanie whipped her head around.

"Why do you hate me?"

"I went online and searched for foods that help boost your immune system."

Trevor walked back into the room holding two mugs with steam rising up from them.

"Green tea with lemon and a sprinkle of ginger."

Trevor handed the mugs to Melanie and Amanda then went back to the kitchen. Amanda put her mug on the table while Melanie took a sip.

"There's no sugar in here."

"Sugar is bad for you."

"If it's so bad for me why does it taste so good?"

Melanie put her mug down, picked up her fork and started poking around at the salad. Trevor walked back in the room with a plate in each hand. Each plate had a homemade cheeseburger and fries on it. He handed one plate to me and the other to Zack. "How come Traci gets a cheeseburger?"

"Cause she's a self-centered brat."

"Were you born this much of a bitch or is it a skill you developed over time?"

"It wouldn't kill you to eat a salad just once in your life."

"Zack is eating the same thing as me. Why aren't you yelling at him?"

"Zack isn't Melanie's sister. I'd expect you of all people to at least pretend you give a fuck."

She always knew exactly what buttons to push. Before I knew it my fries were in Amanda's hair and her spinach was in mine. Zack was behind Amanda with his arms wrapped around her as she flailed erratically. Melanie stood in in front of Amanda trying to calm her down.

I stormed out of the room and as I stepped into the kitchen I bumped into Trevor causing him to drop his bowl, scattering salad all over the floor and spilling the tea onto his shirt.

"Sorry."

"It's alright."

I leaned back against the wall and covered my face with my hands. After a few deep breaths I looked up to see Trevor finish sweeping up the food.

"Everyone's acting like Melanie's gonna die."

"She has cancer."

"That's not a guarantee she's gonna die."

"It's not a guarantee she'll live either."

"Why is this so easy for all of you? I don't want to think about my sister dying. I can't imagine a world without Melanie in it."

Trevor looked in the living room.

"What's the alternative? If we pretend that it's not happening and do nothing, then her death does become a guarantee."

I tried my best to choke back the tears but I couldn't hold them in. Trevor walked over and placed a hand on my shoulder.

"Even if we fight tooth and nail there's no guarantee we can save her. But this is Melanie we're talking about. It's worth trying."

Trevor wrapped his arms around me and held me tight. After crying onto his chest for a few seconds I heard a tapping on the doorframe and turned my head to see Melanie standing in the doorway.

"Zack took Amanda for a drive to clear her head. I came to get the broom but I heard you talking about me and didn't want to interrupt."

I ran over to Melanie and threw my arms around her, squeezing as tight as I could.

"I love you."

"I know baby. I love you too."

We stayed there for a few minutes holding each other and crying while Trevor cleaned the living room.

Forever. Amen

CHAPTER 5

Amanda

The older I get the more I notice my body changing. My metabolism keeps getting slower. There was a time when I could eat nothing but burgers and pizza and couldn't gain a pound if I tried. Now I eat a slice of cake and my pants feel like they're trying to strangle me.

Mornings are the worst. Ten years ago I could wake up with a huge hangover and still manage to slide right out of bed. Nowadays I can go to bed early, get a good eight hours of sleep and it still takes me a while to get on my feet.

My alarm went off and I let it ring for a few minutes before I gathered the strength to lift my hands and turn it off. I held the phone to my face to check the time and felt a groan escape my throat. I dropped my face back onto the pillow and took a deep breath before pushing myself up and sliding my legs out from under the covers.

I stood up, stretching my body. There was so much snapping and popping it sounded like a bowl of Rice Krispies. I picked lint out of my belly button as I trudged down the hall to the bathroom. When I tried to open the door the knob wouldn't turn.

"Someone in there?"

No response. I tried the knob again. It still wouldn't budge so I banged on the door.

"I gotta piss."

Still no answer. I pressed my ear to the door and heard faint whimpering.

"Mel?"

After a short pause I heard a soft "yeah" from the other side of the door. I tried to speak in a calming voice.

"Unlock the door."

No answer.

"Mel....please."

After a few seconds I heard a click. I grabbed the knob, took a deep breath and swung the door open. Melanie was standing by the far wall, her nose running and her face stained with tears. I knew I should say something but I couldn't find the right words. That's when Melanie held out her hand. There was a clump of hair in her palm.

"Mel..."

She started bawling. She was trying to say something but I couldn't hear her words clearly. I ran up to her and wrapped my arms around her. As she cried on my shoulder I stroked the top of her head. More loose strands fell with every brush.

Her tears soaked through my shirt as I held her cold, boney, shivering body in my arms. I knew this was a possibility but it still caught me off guard. The doctor warned us about the side effects. Fatigue was an issue before the chemo. Now it's like she can't keep her eyes open for more than two hours a day. After a few weeks vomiting became a part of her daily routine.

I felt so helpless. Her entire body was falling apart and there was nothing I could do to stop it. I stroked her head once more and another clump of hair came out in my hands. As I stared at my hand I realized that, while I couldn't do anything to stop the pain, I could at least do something to make her smile right now. I put my hands on Melanie's shoulders and gently pushed her away.

"I'll be right back."

I ran out of the bathroom and hurried to the kitchen. I opened a utensil drawer and grabbed a pair of scissors. When I walked back into the bathroom there was fear in Melanie's eyes. I reached behind my head and held a clump of hair in front of my face. Melanie's jaw dropped as the scissors made their way through my hair.

"Mandy…you don't have too."

"I know."

I dropped the loose strands of hair and placed the scissors on the ground. I hurried to the bedroom to grab my phone off the nightstand. Actually, I grabbed Melanie's phone first and had to double back for mine. I sent Zack a quick text while walking back to the bathroom.

"I just texted Zack."

"Why?"

"He cuts his own hair. I asked him to swing by and bring his clippers."

"Your boyfriend cuts his own hair?"

"Something about not wanting to pay for something he can do himself. I don't know. It's a guy thing I guess."

I picked up the scissors and handed them to Melanie. I sat on the floor with my back to her and tilted my head back. She cut my hair as close to the scalp as she felt comfortable getting. Then we switched places and I did the same for her.

By the time Zack arrived we'd already lopped off the majority of our hair. We just needed him to finish us off. I sat on the toilet, the lid was down of course, while Zack shaved my head. Melanie sat on the edge of the tub while she and Zack joked about my head being lumpy.

When it was all done Melanie and I stood in front of each other, smiling and laughing as we each rubbed the other's scalps. Then Melanie flung herself at me, wrapping her arms around my neck. I wrapped my arms around her waist and lightly squeezed her as I felt tears drop onto my shoulder.

CHAPTER 6

Melanie

Turns out, shaving your head in winter isn't a great idea. Especially when your immune system is already compromised. Amanda bought two identical beanies with black and white stripes. I only ever took mine off when I bathed.

Those months of chemo felt like endless torture. Not only did it make my body feel bad, it made everyone treat me differently. Amanda wouldn't let me out of her sight for a second. She was worried that I might pass out on a sidewalk somewhere.

I was vomiting multiple times a day. The taste would stay in my mouth even after I brushed my teeth. That alone made it hard to get excited about eating. At Amanda's insistence I managed to shove a little bit of food in my mouth every day. Just enough to avoid death.

Amanda and I were sitting in Dr. Lewis's office. The moment the doctor walked in the room my heart sank. No one's face looks like that when they're delivering good news. I looked at Amanda and I could tell she saw it too. Dr.

Lewis hadn't said a word and I was already on the verge of tears.

He dropped a large file on his desk, pulled out his chair and let out a grunt as he plopped down. He stared at me with solemn eyes.

"There's no easy way to say this."

Amanda grabbed my hand and squeezed.

"Plain English doc."

He took a deep breath and let it out slowly.

"Your body's response to the chemotherapy has been extremely limited. The results are…negligible at best."

"I said English doc."

"Amanda."

"He's here to tell us you're dying. If that's the case, stop beating around the bush. Say it like you would tell a two year old."

He started rubbing his forehead.

"The cancer has been completely unresponsive."

"You're saying the chemo isn't working at all?"

"Honestly, I can't say that for sure. Your cancer hasn't lessened but it hasn't progressed either. It's possible that yours is incredibly aggressive and the chemotherapy has stopped it in its tracks."

"Does that mean she'll have to keep getting treated for the rest of her life?"

"Unfortunately, that's not a possibility. Before we started, we did warn you of the possibility that there could be many adverse side effects. One of those possibilities was damage to your internal organs."

Tears fell out of my eyes. A surge of emotions rushed through me. I wanted to fall to the floor and cry till I passed out. I wanted to scream at the top of my lungs. A small part of me wanted to just die. Let the cancer overtake my body and be done with the nightmare already.

"How many organs are damaged?"

"In your case, we are specifically worried about the liver. The damage is irreversible."

I couldn't hold back any longer. The tears streamed like rivers while I cried out in agony. Amanda wrapped her arms around my shoulders and held tightly. I spent the rest of the conversation crying my eyes out while they discussed my impending fate.

"So, what I'm hearing is...she's dead no matter which route we take."

"It's a bit more complicated than that. But...that is essentially the case."

I felt something on my forehead. I tilted my head up and saw Amanda in tears.

"What are our options?"

The doctor leaned back in his chair.

"That's the good news. In a situation this desperate everything is an option. Essentially, you're free to just throw shit at a wall until something sticks."

"What is your best recommendation?"

The doctor turned his chair around and rose to his feet. He walked forward, stopping to look out the window.

"There are three options that I believe you should choose from. Option one: We throw everything we have at the cancer hoping that Melanie's body survives long enough to eradicate it completely. Then you have transplant surgery to replace all the damaged organs. Option two: You try every homeopathic remedy that you can find and pray for a miracle."

"And the third option."

He turns back to us with watery eyes.

"Option three: We put her in a bed and give her a steady supply of sedatives."

"What good would that do?"

"It'll ease her pain. When she passes, it'll be peaceful."

"Are you saying we should just accept the fact that she's going to die?"

"Of course not. You asked me for options. That is one of them. If you want my personal opinion...If I were in your shoes, I'd fight to the bitter end."

The tears continued streaming down. I couldn't close my mouth but not sound was coming out. It's like I was gasping for air, struggling with each inhale. I got lightheaded; nearly passed out. I desperately clung to Amanda's arm.

"Take all the time you need."

The doctor walked out of the room, closing the door behind him. I fell to my knees and began dry heaving.

CHAPTER 7

Cynthia

It was a cold, sunny afternoon. The cold wouldn't have felt as horrible if it wasn't so damn windy. Driving up to the house I was struck by a thought. Is this still our house? Do I have any claim left? Should I start calling it their house?

The moment Melanie was diagnosed I left and never returned. My friend let me stay at her place. I was too scared to spend time around Melanie. Being around her too often felt like a big risk since both of our immune systems were compromised.

I wouldn't have shown up if Amanda hadn't called an emergency meeting. I was frightened. The last time and emergency meeting was called it was to inform us that Melanie was diagnosed with cancer. From Amanda's tone of voice I knew she didn't have any good news to share. She called the meeting to tell us that Melanie was dying.

Zack's car was in the driveway so I parked by the curb. The moment I stepped out of my car a huge gust of wind nearly knocked me off my feet, chilling me to the bone. I was shivering as I walked up to the front door. As I reached for the doorknob, my heart beating out of my chest, I heard Traci's voice through the door.

"You can't be fucking serious!"

The tone of her voice confirmed my suspicions. No one would be leaving this building without shedding tears. For a moment I considered jumping back in my car and driving away. Then I realized that whatever I avoided today I would still have to face eventually. Might as well hear it now.

I swung the door open to see Amanda and Traci, their brows furrowed and tears on their cheeks, standing in the middle of the room flailing their arms about as they screamed at each other. Zack was off to the side, sitting in a chair with his head down and his fingers interlocked.

"This isn't about you! It's about what's best for Melanie!"

"How is letting her die what's best for her?"

I put my fingers in my mouth and whistled as loud as I could. Everyone turned their heads to me.

"What's going on?"

Traci stomped towards me and angrily pointed at Amanda.

"She's letting Melanie die!"

"If it was my decision I'd go to every corner of the globe finding every single drug and plant I could just hoping for a miracle! But I have no say! This is Melanie's choice!"

"She always listens to you! If anyone on this planet can change her mind it's you!"

"I may be able to influence her but at the end of the day the choice is still hers!"

"I can't accept that! My sister would never choose to die!"

It felt like they were coming dangerously close to throwing punches so I stepped between them. Staring in Amanda's eyes I could see that her intense, burning anger was a front to mask the immense pain she was in. I understood very well the helplessness she was feeling.

I grabbed Amanda's arm and led her to the couch, shoving her onto the cushion. I sat in front of her on the coffee table and held her face in my hands so I could stare in her eyes. She fought desperately to hold the tears back.

"Tell me what happened?"

Amanda sniffled and a couple of tears rolled down her cheeks.

"I could give you a lot of details if you want. But the gist of it is…there's very little hope of Melanie surviving."

"A little hope is better than none."

Traci took a step towards us and I held an open palm out to her.

"I'd like a couple more details sweetie."

Amanda wiped her nose with her forearm.

"The chemo isn't stopping the cancer…but it is destroying Melanie's organs. If we keep doing the chemo, Melanie will die. If we stop doing the chemo, Melanie will die."

"What does Melanie want to do?"

"The doctor says they can put her in a bed and make her comfortable."

A few teardrops fell out of my eyes. I understood why Traci was so upset. I didn't want to consider the possibility that Melanie would actually choose death. As hard as it was for us to hear, it must have been that much harder for Amanda to say.

"You see what I mean? She's letting Melanie die!"

"I would stop her if I could but it's her decision to make."

"Did you even try to talk her out of it? Hell, how do I know you didn't push her into it?"

Amanda jumped to her feet and I jumped up to stand in front of her out of concern that she was about to charge Traci like a rabid bull.

"You're right! How would you know? You're never there! I'm the one taking time off work to take care of her! Driving her to every hospital visit! Holding her hair back every time she vomits! Where the fuck have you been?"

"I'm sorry I can't just sit there watching my sister die! I'm not a cold hearted bitch like you!"

Amanda shoved me to the side and lunged forward. I fell onto the coffee table. Amanda fell on top of Traci and started punching her face. Zack and I ran over and grabbed Amanda. She was kicking and screaming as we dragged her away.

"You think this is easy for me? It's killing me! But she needs me! She's always relied on me! I've been there for every broken bone and every broken heart!"

Traci crawled to the other side of the room. She was wailing uncontrollably as she put her hands on the wall to help push herself up. She brushed the hair off her face and I saw her left eyes was swollen and she had a cut on her lip.

"I've known her longer and loved her stronger! I've been more of a sister to her than you ever have!"

"Fine! Then I hope you catch her cancer and die with her!"

"That's not how cancer works dumbass!"

Traci stormed out the front door slamming it shut behind her. Amanda stopped struggling so Zack and I let go of her. Zack rose to his feet, grabbed his coat and walked out the front door.

"Zack?"

Amanda jumped to her feet and ran after him.

"Zack. Zack!"

I rose to my feet and walked to the doorway. I stood in the doorframe watching the two of them argue in the driveway.

"I can't do this anymore."

"What are you trying to say?"

"I can't handle it. This isn't what I signed up for."

"Nobody wanted this. It's not like we took a vote and agreed that Melanie needs to have cancer. It happened and we're dealing with it."

"I shouldn't have to be dealing with it."

"And I should?"

"She's your cousin, not mine. I wanted to be your boyfriend. I know that means supporting you but right now you're carrying the weight of the world and that's just too much for me. I need a break."

"You're gonna dump me when I need you the most?"

"It's because you need me so much."

Zack got in his car and slammed the door shut.

"Fine. If you leave now don't ever come back. I never wanna see your face again."

As Zack drove away Amanda fell to her knees. I walked to the driveway. By the time I reached her Amanda was down on her hands and knees wailing. I squatted down beside her and placed a hand on her back. She turned her head to me, her face covered in tears and boogers.

"Everything is falling apart."

She threw her arms around my waist, burying her head in my chest. I wrapped my arms around her shoulders and kissed the top of her head. After a few seconds I rose to my feet, lifting her up with me.

I led her back inside. We barely made it through the door before her legs gave out. We collapsed just inside the front door, sitting on the floor with our backs against the wall. I stretched my arm out, barely grabbing the edge of the door with my fingertips.

I slammed it shut, leaned back against the wall, then took in a deep breath and let out an exasperated sigh. Amanda pulled her knees up to her chest. She rested her arms on her knees and her head on her arms. Her wailing reduced to light sobbing.

"Melanie's dying and nobody cares."

"Of course they care sweetie."

"Do they?! Do You? You've been avoiding her, Trevor disappeared, Zack ran away and Traci refuses to accept the truth."

"Everyone deals with death in their own way."

"They're not dealing with it. They're all running away. You're running away. Melanie's running away.

"She's not running away. She's dying."

"But she doesn't have to accept it so easily. She doesn't have to give up."

"Well...now we're getting somewhere."

I put my hands on the ground and pushed myself upright.

"The real issue here is that you're pissed at Melanie, but you can't punch the cancer patient."

Amanda grabs the front of her shirt, lifting it up to wipe her nose.

"How come you're not upset?"

"I am."

"You don't seem too upset to me."

"That's because you're so upset."

"What does that have to do with anything?"

She turned her head and trained her puffy eyes on me. I couldn't help but smile.

"Do you remember when we learned I was HIV positive?"

"Yeah. That barely bothered you either. It seems like nothing ever gets to you."

"That's not true. I was crying myself to sleep every night."

Amanda sniffled and wiped the tears off her face.

"Really?"

I nodded.

"As scared as I was, you were freaking out even more. It was easy to pretend to be strong when I was around you because I knew that's what you needed."

I placed a hand on her back and started rubbing.

"I'm starting to think that attitude might be genetic."

"Well, if that's the case, it must've skipped Traci."

I chuckled.

"No it didn't. She's the baby of the bunch. We've always looked after her. She's never had to look after us."

Using my arm I hooked her neck and pulled her close, resting my head on top of hers. For a moment, I felt slightly relieved. My baby sister still needed me. My job as big sister wasn't done yet.

"Mandy…we have to start telling everyone."

"Melanie said she didn't want any of our relatives to know."

"She didn't want them to know she was fighting cancer because she didn't want them to worry for no reason. If she doesn't intend to keep fighting then we have a reason to tell them. They deserve the chance to say goodbye."

CHAPTER 8

Amanda

Spreading word of Melanie's impending death was the most difficult task I've ever had to complete. I sent emails and letters, made phone calls and posted on every social media I had. I made sure that every family member, coworker and classmate knew that this was their last chance to see her face.

Over the next few weeks we endured an endless parade of well-wishers journeying from near and far. Every living relative, every friend Melanie made in her life, paid a visit to her hospital room.

Though they came to deliver their final goodbyes the majority of them couldn't bring themselves to actually say those words. Many of them presented Melanie with home remedies and the names of specialist from around the world. Every single one of them promised to keep her in their prayers.

Nearly every single relative, the moment they were done with Melanie, would leave the room and tell me in their loudest voice every single mistake I made.

They'd tell me I shouldn't let Melanie give up. I'd tell them I was just respecting her wishes. They'd tell me I should've called them sooner. Maybe they could've convinced her to keep fighting. The first few times, I had this argument with tears in my eyes. After a while it just became part of the routine.

Cynthia only dropped by the hospital once. She confided in me that it was difficult to see Melanie going through this. It forced her to confront her own potential mortality. Still, she made sure to visit because she knew Melanie wanted to see her.

That's the one positive about this situation. Melanie could get everyone who cared about her to do anything she ask. It's impossible to say no to the request of a dying woman. That's why when Melanie told me to apologize to Traci I didn't hesitate.

Apologizing has never been easy for me. Especially when I'm not wrong. For Melanie's sake, I had to swallow my pride. Once Traci and I cleared the air we began taking turns watching over Melanie, supporting each other in our support of her.

When we first checked her into the hospital Melanie was all smiles as usual. I could tell she was putting on a brave face to keep us from feeling sad. Cynthia was right. It is genetic.

As the days turned to weeks the depression set in. The doctor warned us that the emotional damage might take more of a toll than the physical pain. It reached a point where Melanie refused to eat anymore. All she would say is that she wasn't hungry. The doctor examined her and said there was nothing physically wrong. In fact, Melanie was incredibly malnourished. The doctor encouraged her to eat more.

I did everything I could, short of shoving the food down her throat. It wasn't until Traci broke down in tears that we finally got through to Melanie. She started forcing herself to eat at least a little bit of every meal we bring her.

Even though we accepted the fact that Melanie was dying it still wasn't easy to watch it happening. The more time that passed the more tears we all shed. Anytime I was home I cried myself to sleep. Sometimes when I stayed at the hospital I'd wake up in the middle of the night to the sound of Melanie's muffled sobs.

Most nights I pretended not to notice. She obviously didn't want us to know just how bad she was hurting. She'd always wait for us to leave or fall asleep. For some reason, that night was different. My best friend was suffering. I couldn't sit there doing nothing. If there was any way for me to ease her pain I had to try.

I set the blanket aside, rose out of my chair and tiptoed over to her bed. When I placed my hand on her shoulder she jerked her head towards me. I caught her off guard. She stopped crying for a brief second, then burst into tears once more as she flung herself into my arms.

I stood there with my arms wrapped around her, holding her tightly until her tears dried up. I slid my hand under my shirt and wiped her face clean. She sniffled, swallowed a lump in her throat, then looked up at me with sad eyes.

"I'm dying."

Her words cut through me like a knife made of ice stabbing right through my heart.

"I know."

What else could I say? There's no lie I could tell that would ease her suffering.

"It's happening soon."

Anger. Sadness. Fear. Concern. Maybe even a little bit of relief. Enormous guilt for feeling relieved. I couldn't stop the flood of emotions. I was feeling everything all at once.

"What makes you so sure?"

She shrugs and shakes her head.

"I don't know. It's just that...my body feels like it's about ready to give out."

I placed a hand on top of her head.

"What can I do?"

"I want to see Trevor."

The words shocked and appalled don't come close to describing my feelings. I would never have guessed that those would be the words to leave her mouth in that moment. He can't be the reason she cried every night. Is this really her dying wish?

"I haven't seen him in months. I want to say goodbye."

Well, that does make sense. Still, it bothered me to hear her beg for a guy that abandoned her when she needed him the most. No one told him not to come. He decided all on his own to stop showing up. So did Zack. Even Cynthia and Traci disappeared for a while. Everyone ran away except me. Does that make me strong or just a martyr?

Unfortunately, as much as I disagreed with her request, someone I love was crying in my arms. She was on the brink of death and there was only one thing she wanted. Actually…there might be one other thing she desired even more. I'm sure she wished she could be healthy again. Since I couldn't get rid of her cancer, there was only one final favor I could do for her.

Forever. Amen

CHAPTER 9

Trevor

I was looking forward to the end of winter. The temperature rose for a few days before a cold front moved in. Our local meteorologist said it would be another few weeks before things heated up again.

"Sure you don't need a ride Trevor?"

"I'm good. Thanks."

I pulled up the zipper on my light grey cotton jacket and threw the hood over my head. When I stepped out the door the sunlight was somewhat blinding. A cold wind chilled me to the bone. I shoved my shivering hands in the jacket pockets and started down the street.

You know that song that Belle sings at the beginning of Beauty and the Beast? Some days that's what the walk home feels like. Same three people sitting at the bus stop, waiting for the twenty which is always fifteen minutes late. That day, I saw something different. A block away, on the other side of Martin Street, stood Amanda with folded arms and a furrowed brow.

She was bundled up tight, wearing nothing but black. Her jacket, gloves, boots and scarf...all black. The white stripes on her beanie the only variance in her outfit. Her face was devoid of any makeup. Her skin looked dry. Her lips were chapped. Had she been out here for a while? Why?

Our eyes locked. Her gaze answered all my questions. She was here for me. When someone who despises you so strongly actively seeks you out there are only a few explanations that make sense. My heart sank. I knew this would happen. I wasn't ready to hear it so soon.

She rushed across the street, heading straight for me. I hurried to the corner and pushed the button for the crosswalk. Amanda was getting closer with each step. If traffic were lighter I would've weaved through the cars like a live action game of Frogger. The idea of talking to Amanda was only slightly less horrifying than the prospect of getting flattened by a truck.

"Trevor."

I closed my eyes and lightly banged my head against the pole. I mumbled some words of encouragement to myself before turning to face Amanda. Her breathing was heavy. There were bags under her eyes. From the concaving of her cheeks I got the impression that if she were to disrobe I'd be able to see the outline of every bone and organ in her body.

She had a look in her eyes. Could it be fear? How is it possible that someone who inspires so much anxiety in others could be trembling before me? They say wild animals are more afraid of you than you are of them.

"Hey."

"Hey."

"It's been a while."

"Yeah."

"Haven't seen you in months."

"I've been around."

"Not around us. Not around Melanie."

I turned my head. I couldn't bear to look in her eyes. The icy glare sent shivers down my spine. I felt like a child about to be lectured by my mother. She's not angry, just disappointed.

"I've been busy."

"Too busy to send even one text?"

"Winter is our busiest season of the year."

"Don't give me that bullshit. We've all got lives to live and bills to pay but when someone you care about is struggling you make time to be there for them!"

"Don't you dare say I don't care about her!"

"You aren't acting like you do!"

My heart was racing. I felt lightheaded. I was trying my best to hold it in but I couldn't stop the tears from falling.

"Maybe I don't visit because I care! Maybe I can't stand to just sit there watching her die knowing there's not a single fucking thing I can do about it!"

I covered my face with my hands trying to hide the waterfalls bursting from my eyes. My legs started feeling weak so I leaned back against the pole. The metal was so cold it penetrated every layer of clothing I had.

"This hasn't been easy for me either. I can't eat. I can't sleep. My heart feels like it's been torn to shreds. But as painful as it is to sit by and watch her slowly slip away, I know it would be even more painful for Melanie if she was forced to go through this alone."

I reached down to grab my knees. I was having trouble catching my breath between sobs. I looked at Amanda. Her legs were shaking like two twigs trying to hold the weight of an elephant.

"Are you cold?"

"A little."

"Maybe we should get inside."

"Maybe we should go to the hospital."

I chortled and roll my eyes. This woman's like a heat seeking missile. Unyielding in the pursuit of her target.

"You do understand that she's dying don't you?"

"Isn't that what this entire conversation's been about?"

"This could be your last chance to see her. Why wouldn't you want to take advantage of the opportunity?"

"You wouldn't understand."

"Explain it to me."

My mouth was dry and my throat was sore. I licked my lips and swallowed what little saliva I had. I raised my head to look Amanda in the eyes. Her features softened. She never seemed so gentle before. For better or worse, Amanda was determined to get me into that hospital room.

"It hurts. Everything…hurts. Every time I think about her it just…hurts. It hurts to know that she'll be gone soon. That I'll never see her smile again. That I'll never hear her laugh again. It just…hurts."

"I know it hurts. I'm hurting too. But think about it Trevor. How long has it been since you last saw her smile? How many months ago did you last hear her laugh? The way you're acting now…it's like she's already dead."

The moment she said those words all the strength left my body and I collapsed. It must have been quite the sight for those passing by. Me sitting on the ground with my back to the pole, crying like a baby with my knees pulled up to my chest. Amanda stepped forward and squatted down, her face only inches from mine.

"This has been hard on everyone. Especially Melanie."

She put a hand underneath my chin and lifted my head up.

"But right now, she is still alive. And she wants to see you."

I looked at Amanda's face and saw tears streaming down her cheeks. No matter our differences there is at least one thing we have in common. We were both in a lot of pain.

Forever. Amen

CHAPTER 10

Melanie

I always knew I would die someday. It's the inevitable end to every life. I just didn't think it would happen so soon. I was supposed to be in my 80s with a bunch of grandkids. Instead, I die unmarried with no kids and no pictures of the family vacation to Italy. It's not fair.

When I was first diagnosed I tried to stay optimistic. Then it became an undeniable fact that my body would shut down and I'd find out for sure whether or not heaven was real. What's the right way to feel when you know you could be hours away from death? Sadness? Anger? Excitement? Some days it was all of the above.

There's nothing scarier than knowing that every time I close my eyes I might never open them again. Every morning I woke up feeling a strange blend of relief and disappointment. There were days when the pain was so unbearable that I couldn't wait for it to be over.

Worst of all, I felt so guilty. I love Amanda and Traci so dearly. I wouldn't have survived without them. I hated seeing them in pain. Every time they walked through the door with puffy red eyes I found myself wishing neither of them gave a shit about me.

The people I love kept shedding tears because of me. While the prospect of my death did scare me, I worried even more about them. I want the people I love to live with smiles on their faces. The possibility that for the rest of their lives they'd be sad every time they thought of me brought me immeasurable pain.

Trevor once told me that he hates hospitals. He's never stepped foot in one unless it was absolutely necessary. That's the main reason I told Melanie I wanted to see him. I was forcing her to leave. I knew she wouldn't walk back in the room without him. I didn't want her to be there when I died.

I should've known that, while Trevor's stubbornness did rival hers, no one in this world was quite as forceful as Amanda. She always accomplished every goal she set for herself.

I was laying in my hospital bed, staring out the window, wondering how many days I had left before I passed away. When the door swung open I didn't even turn my head. The majority of times when that door opened the person who steps through is either Traci, Amanda or a nurse.

I realized fairly quickly that someone new had stepped through the door. The footsteps were heavier. So was the breathing. The hand that was placed on top of mine was larger and rougher than any I'd felt in a while.

I'd been having trouble feeling happy. I tried my best to force a smile whenever people were around but most days I could only muster a minor smirk at best. When I turned my head and saw Trevor's face a real smile spread across my face for the first time in weeks.

I was angry. He ignored me for months while I suffered. Despite that, I was overjoyed to see his face again after all this time away. I've missed you. Those are the only words I wanted to say.

"Hey."

"Hey."

How pathetic is that? After months of not seeing each other the most we could muster was one word each. That one word was enough to bring tears to my eyes.

"How are you?"

"I've been better."

"You've looked better."

"Look who's talking."

We both chuckled. I squeeze his hand. I felt a sudden urge and struggled to lift myself upright. It's hard to believe how much effort it took just to sit up straight. It was painful.

I held my arms up. Trevor leaned forward. I'd almost forgotten how great it felt to be wrapped in the warmth and comfort of his arms.

"I've missed you."

"I've missed you too."

He was trembling. I leaned back to look at him. Tears were streaming down his face. I put my hands on his cheeks and stared into his eyes.

"What's wrong?"

"You're dying."

"I know."

"Why aren't you more upset about this?"

"I was. I've had time to cope."

"I'm sorry it took me so long. I was just so scared."

"I know. I forgive you."

He said something else but I couldn't understand it through the sobbing.

"Trevor...I'm dying. That scares me. But I'm even more scared of what's gonna to happen to you."

He looks at me, confused.

"I'm leaving behind people I care about."

I glanced over at Amanda. She was standing in the doorway, her back leaning against the frame, silently staring at us with a solemn expression.

"People who rely on me."

I turned back to Trevor and tears began streaming down my face. I'd been holding back but I ran out of strength.

"I need you to do me a favor. I need you to take care of Amanda for me. She's gonna need someone to take care of her when I'm gone. She's not as strong as she wants everyone to believe."

He swallowed a lump in his throat and nodded twice. I felt all the strength leaving my body and laid back down. When my head touched the pillow my eyes closed almost immediately. Then Trevor grabbed my hand. I opened my eyes and smiled at him.

"Stay with me."

"I'm never gonna leave your side again."

"What about when I leave you?"

"You're never gonna leave."

He pointed a finger at his head.

"You'll always be right here…"

He grabbed my hand and put it on his chest. I felt his heart pounding.

"…and right here."

A wide smile spread across my face as my eyes filled with water. Amanda turned her back to me. Her forearm resting against the wall; her forehead resting on her arm. I didn't have to see the tears to know she was crying.

What a sight we must've been. Amanda somehow managing to bawl her eyes out without making a single sound. Trevor and I staring at each other with smiles on our faces and tears streaming down our cheeks.

Forever. Amen

CHAPTER 11

Amanda

For the next three days Trevor never left Melanie's bedside. When visiting hours were over the nurses told us only family could stay. We said he was Melanie's husband. They knew we were lying. They let him stay anyway.

Every time Melanie fell asleep he was holding her hand. Every time she woke up her hand was still nestled inside of his. He was there for every smile and every tear she cried.

One morning I walked into the room and he was sitting by her bed, holding her hand in his, gently stroking her fingers. His face was stained with tears. Her skin was pale. All the machines attached to her were turned off.

"2:36 am."

I fell to my knees and cried. I knew this day would come. I was prepared for it. It was still the worst feeling I've ever experienced in my life. I felt like I might shatter to pieces.

Trevor got on his knees and wrapped his arms around me. He pulled me close and held me tight. I grabbed onto his shirt and twisted it. I cried out in pain as I bawled uncontrollably.

My life after that was a blur. It felt like I was moving in slow motion while the world kept spinning normally around me. How could everyone move on with their lives as if nothing happened? How could I pretend that my heart hasn't been ripped out? Her memories were haunting me every moment. Every time I closed my eyes I saw her face. Every time I opened them tears fall.

Melanie's body was frozen until the funeral. I was put in charge of planning it but I wouldn't have made any progress if Cynthia and Trevor weren't helping me. I started understanding why Melanie thought so highly of Trevor. He's incredibly caring and reliable.

He stayed with me every step of the way. When I was informing all our friends and family of Melanie's death he was there to hold my hand. When I was so depressed that I couldn't even crawl out of bed he would carry me to the table and put food in front of me.

The day of the funeral he was the one to give a speech for Melanie. The rest of us couldn't choke back the tears long enough to get a single word out. He stood in front of everyone, trembling like a zebra staring down a pride of lions.

"I don't feel comfortable being the one to give this speech. The majority of people here knew Melanie much longer than I did. I don't have to tell you how amazing she was. How her smile lit up the room. That when she looked at you...it felt like you might be the only person in the world. And when she believed in you, you knew you could do anything.

I don't have to tell you what you already know. So I'll keep my message as short as possible. Melanie is dead...but she's not gone. She still exist in every one of us. As long as you remember her, she will always be alive. So I beg of you, please, remember her. Remember every smile. Remember every tear. Those of you who knew Melanie long enough that you actually managed to piss her off, please remember her scowl.

Remember her. Keep her in your hearts and in your minds. I'm not a religious person...but from now until the day I die, I will be. Today, I say my first prayer. God, if you really are up there, please keep Melanie by your side. Keep her safe...and make sure she smiles forever. Amen."

Trevor was the only one who made it through his speech without crying. As soon as he said the final word the tears begin flowing as strongly out of his eyes as they were ours.

Trevor was one of the pallbearers when we took Melanie's coffin to her gravesite. He stood by my side as we watched it lowered into the ground. Three hours later, once the ground had been smoothed over and everyone else left, he was still there.

The air got colder. I folded my arms and started rubbing them. I had to keep my mouth shut to keep my teeth from chattering.

"Why are you still here?"

"Probably the same reason as you."

"Then can you tell me why I'm here?"

"You don't know?"

"Not really. All I know is...I can't bring myself to walk away."

"Cause you know that the moment you leave, she's officially gone."

The moment he said that the tears started falling again. I didn't understand how I could keep crying. It felt like I hadn't stopped since Melanie died. How did my body even have that much water in it?

"Yeah. I guess you're right."

He placed a hand on my shoulder. His grip was strong yet his touch was gentle and comforting. I felt a sensation that could only be described as butterflies in my stomach. Then a wave of guilt hit me.

"If I stayed here till the sun finished setting, would you stay with me?"

"I'd stand here with you till the sun rose."

"Why!"

My head jerked in his direction. I was scowling at him. I don't know why. I was feeling so many conflicting emotions in that moment. I couldn't keep my thoughts straight.

"Melanie told me to take care of you. I plan to keep my promise."

I cold wind blew. Trevor must've seen me shivering because he took off his jacket and held it out to me. I lunged forward and wrapped my arms around his body, burying my face in his chest and crying. He placed the jacket on my back then wrapped his arms around me.

Other Books by Nathan Lyle Cunningham

Series #1 | TOXIC – *Before the Beginning*

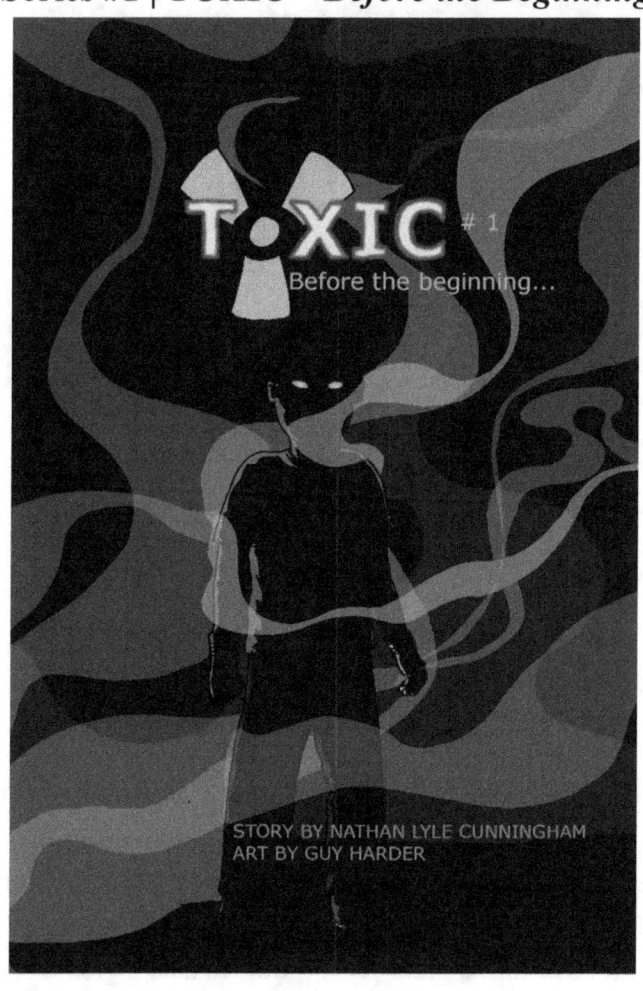

Series #2 | TOXIC

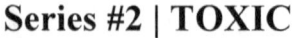

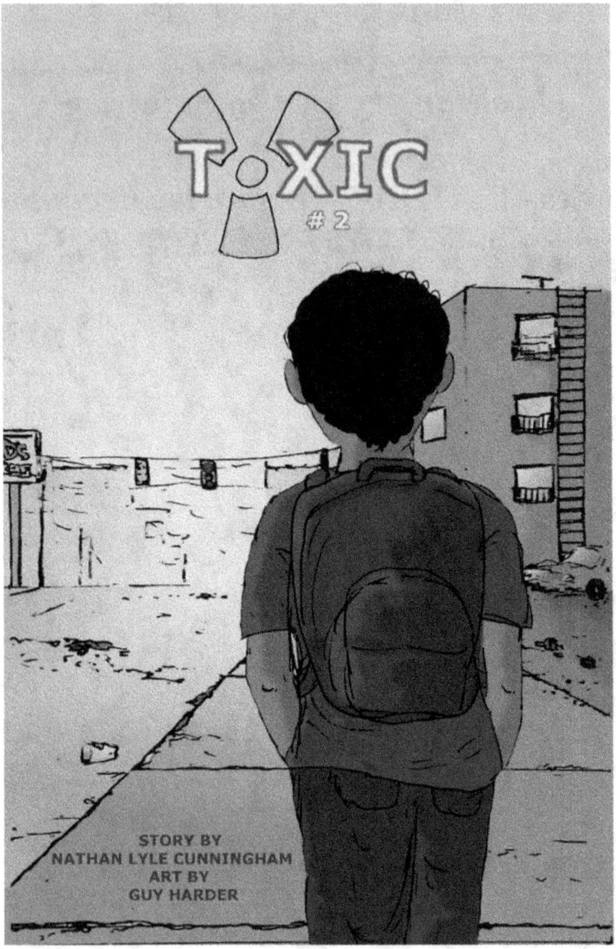

COMIC BOOK SERIES about Oscar Mireles, a boy from a town that was overrun with radiation. While more than half the town died somehow Oscar was infused with radiation. An accident that took many lives gave Oscar the power to save some. It gave him a great power, but it's also a great curse.

Other Books by Nathan Lyle Cunningham

Everything Is Impossible

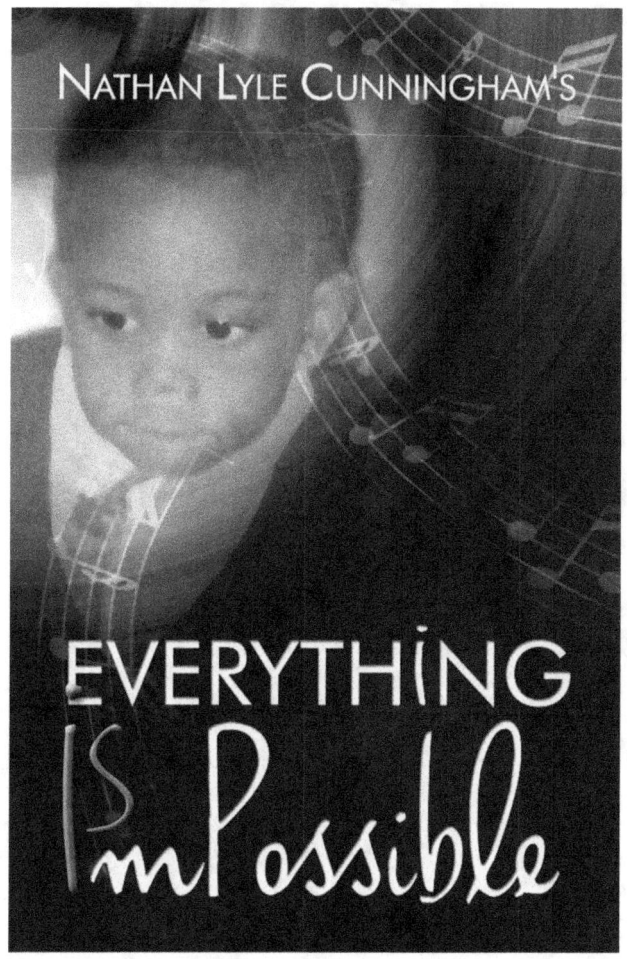

I was physically abused at home. I was picked on and beaten up at school. I tried to kill myself every year of high school. I ran away as a teenager. I was homeless for two years. Somewhere in the middle of all this I found a dream worth chasing. This is the story of my life in my own words.

Nathan Lyle Cunningham
www.YouTube.com/NathanLyleOfficial
www.Twitter.com/NathanLyle

www.ingramcontent.com/pod-product-compliance
Lightning Source LLC
Chambersburg PA
CBHW071912070526
44583CB00016B/1958